Copyright © 2021 by Alexandra Bella, RDN

Contents

A gastric bypass diet helps people who are recovering from sleeve gastrectomy and from gastric bypass surgery.

The gastric bypass diet is designed to:

Allow your stomach to heal without being stretched by the food you eat

Get you used to eating the smaller amounts of food that your smaller stomach can comfortably and safely digest

Help you lose weight and avoid gaining weight

Avoid side effects and complications from the surgery.

DELECTABLE GASTRIC BYPASS DIET RECIPES

1. Deep-Fried Tilapia

Prep: 10 mins

Cook: 10 mins

Total: 20 mins

Servings: 10

Ingredients

- 10 (4 ounce) fillets tilapia
- salt and ground black pepper to taste
- ⅓ cup all-purpose flour
- 1 cup buttermilk
- 1 egg
- ½ cup all-purpose flour
- ½ cup yellow cornmeal
- 2 tablespoons seafood seasoning
- ½ teaspoon baking powder
- ½ teaspoon baking soda
- vegetable oil for frying

Directions

1. Season fillets with salt and pepper. Dust with 1/3 cup of flour.
2. Beat buttermilk and egg in a bowl. Combine remaining flour, cornmeal, seafood seasoning, baking powder, and baking soda in another bowl. Dip all flour-dusted fillets into egg mixture, then into seasoned flour mixture.

3. Heat oil over medium-high heat in a large frying pan or deep fryer. Fry fillets, working in batches if needed, until golden, about 2 minutes on each side. Season again with salt as soon as your take them out of the pan or fryer.

Prep: 5 mins

Cook: 7 mins

Total: 12 mins

Servings: 8

Ingredients

- 1 ¼ cups cornmeal
- 2 ½ cups water
- ½ teaspoon salt

Directions

1. Mix together cornmeal, water, and salt in a medium saucepan. Cook over medium heat, stirring frequently, until mixture thickens, about 5 to 7 minutes.
2. If using as cereal, spoon mush into bowls and serve with milk and sugar, if desired. If frying, pour mixture into a loaf pan and chill completely. Remove from pan, cut into slices, and fry in a small amount of oil over medium-high heat until browned on both sides. Serve with sauce of your choice.

Prep: 15 mins

Cook: 20 mins

Total: 35 mins

Servings: 6

Ingredients

- ⅓ cup vegetable oil for frying
- 1 ½ cups cornmeal
- ½ cup all-purpose flour
- 1 tablespoon seasoned salt
- ½ tablespoon lemon pepper
- 1 tablespoon kosher salt
- ½ teaspoon ground white pepper
- 3 eggs
- 6 salmon fillets, or to taste

Directions

1. Heat oil to 350 degrees F (175 degrees C) in a cast iron skillet over medium heat.
2. Whisk cornmeal, flour, seasoned salt, lemon pepper, kosher salt, and white pepper together in a medium bowl.
3. Crack eggs into a separate bowl; beat about 10 seconds. Dip salmon fillet into the eggs and coat completely. Dredge salmon in the cornmeal mixture to cover completely. Shake off excess.
4. Lower salmon carefully into the hot oil in batches of 2 or 3. Fry, flipping halfway, until a golden brown crust forms, 8 to 10 minutes. Transfer to a plate lined with 3

to 4 sheets of paper towels to drain. Repeat with remaining salmon.

Prep: 15 mins

Cook: 30 mins

Total: 45 mins

Servings: 18

Yield: 3 dozen

Ingredients

- ¾ cup butter, softened
- ¾ cup white sugar
- 1 egg
- 1 ½ cups all-purpose flour
- ½ cup cornmeal
- 1 teaspoon baking powder
- ¼ teaspoon salt
- 1 teaspoon vanilla extract
- ½ cup raisins

Directions

1. In a large bowl, blend butter and sugar until creamy. Add egg and beat well.
2. In another bowl, stir together flour, cornmeal, baking powder and salt; gradually add to butter mixture. Add vanilla and blend thoroughly. Stir in the optional raisins.
3. Form dough into ball, wrap tightly in plastic wrap, and chill until firm, about 1 hour.
4. Roll out dough on well-floured board to 1/4 inch thickness. Cut with cookie cutters (2 1/2 inches in

diameter) and place 1 inch apart on lightly greased cookie sheet.

5. Bake in 350 degree F (175 degrees C) oven for 10-12 minutes or until edges are golden. Store in airtight container.

Prep: 20 mins

Cook: 20 mins

Total: 40 mins

Servings: 24

Ingredients

- peanut or corn oil for frying
- ¾ cup self-rising flour
- ½ cup self-rising cornmeal mix
- ¼ cup sugar
- ½ teaspoon ground cinnamon
- ¼ teaspoon freshly grated nutmeg
- 1 egg
- ½ cup buttermilk
- 1 tablespoon cinnamon
- ½ cup sugar

Directions

1. Heat oil in deep-fryer to 375 degrees F (190 degrees C).
2. In a bowl, combine the flour, cornmeal mix, sugar, cinnamon, and nutmeg. In a separate bowl, beat the egg together with the buttermilk. Gradually add the egg mixture to the dry ingredients, stirring with a fork or whisk until only slightly lumpy. Be careful not to overmix.
3. Carefully drop batter by the rounded teaspoonful into hot oil, and fry until golden brown. Drain and cool on a paper towel-lined plate. Roll balls in a small amount of

cinnamon mixed with sugar, if desired, or just enjoy plain.

Active: 30 mins

Total: 45 mins

Servings: 4

Ingredients

- 3 tablespoons low-fat mayonnaise
- 1 teaspoon chili powder
- 2 medium sweet potatoes, peeled and cut into 1-inch cubes
- 4 teaspoons olive oil, divided
- ½ teaspoon salt, divided
- ¼ teaspoon ground pepper, divided
- 4 cups broccoli florets (8 oz.; 1 medium crown)
- 1 ¼ pounds salmon fillet, cut into 4 portions
- 2 limes, 1 zested and juiced, 1 cut into wedges for serving
- ¼ cup crumbled feta or cotija cheese
- ½ cup chopped fresh cilantro

Directions

1. Preheat oven to 425 degrees F. Line a large rimmed baking sheet with foil and coat with cooking spray.
2. Combine mayonnaise and chili powder in a small bowl. Set aside.
3. Toss sweet potatoes with 2 tsp. oil, 1/4 tsp. salt, and 1/8 tsp. pepper in a medium bowl. Spread on the prepared baking sheet. Roast for 15 minutes.
4. Meanwhile, toss broccoli with the remaining 2 tsp. oil, 1/4 tsp. salt, and 1/8 tsp. pepper in the same bowl.

Remove the baking sheet from oven. Stir the sweet potatoes and move them to the sides of the pan. Arrange salmon in the center of the pan and spread the broccoli on either side, among the sweet potatoes. Spread 2 Tbsp. of the mayonnaise mixture over the salmon. Bake until the sweet potatoes are tender and the salmon flakes easily with a fork, about 15 minutes.

5. Meanwhile, add lime zest and lime juice to the remaining 1 Tbsp. mayonnaise; mix well.

6. Divide the salmon among 4 plates and top with cheese and cilantro. Divide the sweet potatoes and broccoli among the plates and drizzle with the lime-mayonnaise sauce. Serve with lime wedges and any remaining sauce.

Active: 10 mins

Total: 40 mins

Servings: 4

Ingredients

- 1 pound baby Yukon Gold potatoes, halved
- 2 tablespoons extra-virgin olive oil, divided
- ¾ teaspoon salt, divided
- ½ teaspoon ground pepper, divided
- 12 ounces asparagus, trimmed
- 2 tablespoons melted butter
- 1 tablespoon lemon juice
- 2 cloves garlic, minced
- 1 ¼ pounds salmon fillet, skinned and cut into 4 portions
- Chopped parsley for garnish

Directions

1. Preheat oven to 400 degrees F. Toss potatoes, 1 tablespoon oil, 1/4 teaspoon salt and 1/8 teaspoon pepper together in a medium bowl. Spread in an even layer on a large rimmed baking sheet. Roast until starting to soften and brown, about 15 minutes.
2. Meanwhile, toss asparagus with the remaining 1 tablespoon oil, 1/8 teaspoon salt and 1/8 teaspoon pepper in the medium bowl. Combine butter, lemon juice, garlic, 1/4 teaspoon salt and the remaining 1/4 teaspoon pepper in a small bowl.

3. Sprinkle salmon with the remaining 1/8 teaspoon salt. Move the potatoes to one side of the pan. Place the salmon in the center of the pan; drizzle with the butter mixture. Spread the asparagus on the empty side of the pan. Roast until the salmon is just cooked through and the vegetables are tender, 10 to 12 minutes. Garnish with parsley.

Total: 50 mins

Servings: 6

Ingredients

ADOBO-RUBBED FISH

- 4 teaspoons chili powder, preferably made with New Mexico or ancho chiles
- 2 tablespoons lime juice
- 2 tablespoons extra-virgin olive oil
- 1 teaspoon ground cumin
- 1 teaspoon onion powder
- 1 teaspoon garlic powder
- 1 teaspoon salt
- ½ teaspoon freshly ground pepper
- 2 pounds mahi-mahi or Pacific halibut, 1/2-3/4 inch thick, skinned and cut into 4 portions

COLESLAW

- ¼ cup reduced-fat sour cream
- ¼ cup low-fat mayonnaise
- 2 tablespoons chopped fresh cilantro
- 1 teaspoon lime zest
- 2 tablespoons lime juice
- 1 teaspoon sugar
- ⅛ teaspoon salt

FRESHLY GROUND PEPPER

- 3 cups finely shredded red or green cabbage
- 12 corn tortillas, warmed

Directions

1. To prepare fish: Combine chili powder, lime juice, oil, cumin, onion powder, garlic powder, salt and pepper in a small bowl. Rub adobo rub all over fish. Let stand 20 to 30 minutes for the fish to absorb the flavor.
2. To prepare coleslaw: Combine sour cream, mayonnaise, cilantro, lime zest, lime juice, sugar, salt and pepper in a medium bowl; mix until smooth and creamy. Add cabbage and toss to combine. Refrigerate until ready to use.
3. Preheat grill to medium-high.
4. Oil the grill rack
5. or use a grilling basket. Grill the fish until it is cooked through and easily flakes with a fork, 3 to 5 minutes per side. Transfer the fish to a platter and separate into large chunks.
6. Serve the tacos family-style by passing the fish, tortillas, coleslaw and taco garnishes separately.

Total: 30 mins

Servings: 4

Ingredients

- 1 ¼ pounds wild salmon, skinned and cut into 4 portions
- 3 tablespoons extra-virgin olive oil, divided
- 1 tablespoon minced garlic
- ¾ teaspoon salt
- 2 tablespoons mayonnaise
- 2 teaspoons whole-grain mustard
- ½ teaspoon ground pepper, divided
- 12 ounces pretrimmed haricots verts or thin green beans, cut into thirds
- 1 small lemon, zested and cut into 4 wedges
- 2 tablespoons pine nuts
- 1 8-ounce package precooked brown rice
- 2 tablespoons water
- Chopped fresh parsley for garnish

Directions

1. Preheat oven to 425 degrees F. Line a rimmed baking sheet with foil or parchment paper.
2. Brush salmon with 1 tablespoon oil and place on the prepared baking sheet. Mash garlic and salt into a paste with the side of a chef's knife or a fork. Combine a scant 1 teaspoon of the garlic paste in a small bowl with mayonnaise, mustard and 1/4 teaspoon pepper. Spread the mixture on top of the fish.

3. Roast the salmon until it flakes easily with a fork in the thickest part, 6 to 8 minutes per inch of thickness.

4. Meanwhile, heat the remaining 2 tablespoons oil in a large skillet over medium-high heat. Add green beans, lemon zest, pine nuts, the remaining garlic paste and 1/4 teaspoon pepper; cook, stirring, until the beans are just tender, 2 to 4 minutes. Reduce heat to medium. Add rice and water and cook, stirring, until hot, 2 to 3 minutes more.

5. Sprinkle the salmon with parsley, if desired, and serve with the green bean pilaf and lemon wedges.

Active: 35 mins

Total: 55 mins

Servings: 4

Ingredients

- 1 pound fingerling potatoes, halved lengthwise
- 2 tablespoons olive oil
- 5 garlic cloves, coarsely chopped
- ½ teaspoon sea salt
- ½ teaspoon freshly ground black pepper
- 4 5 to 6-ounce fresh or frozen skinless salmon fillets
- 2 medium red, yellow and/or orange sweet peppers, cut into rings
- 2 cups cherry tomatoes
- 1 ½ cups chopped fresh parsley (1 bunch)
- ¼ cup pitted kalamata olives, halved
- ¼ cup finely snipped fresh oregano or 1 Tbsp. dried oregano, crushed
- 1 lemon

Directions

1. Preheat oven to 425 degrees F. Place potatoes in a large bowl. Drizzle with 1 Tbsp. of the oil and sprinkle with garlic and 1/8 tsp. of the salt and black pepper; toss to coat. Transfer to a 15x10-inch baking pan; cover with foil. Roast 30 minutes.
2. Meanwhile, thaw salmon, if frozen. Combine, in the same bowl, sweet peppers, tomatoes, parsley, olives,

oregano and 1/8 tsp. of the salt and black pepper. Drizzle with remaining 1 Tbsp. oil; toss to coat.

3. Rinse salmon; pat dry. Sprinkle with remaining 1/4 tsp. salt and black pepper. Spoon sweet pepper mixture over potatoes and top with salmon. Roast, uncovered, 10 minutes more or just until salmon flakes.

4. Remove zest from lemon. Squeeze juice from lemon over salmon and vegetables. Sprinkle with zest.

Prep: 15 mins

Cook: 40 mins

Total: 55 mins

Servings: 9

Ingredients

- ½ cup packed light brown sugar
- 1 cup all-purpose flour
- ¼ teaspoon baking soda
- ⅛ teaspoon salt
- 1 cup rolled oats
- ½ cup butter, softened
- ¾ cup seedless raspberry jam

Directions

1. Preheat oven to 350 degrees F (175 degrees C). Grease one 8 inch square pan, and line with greased foil.
2. Combine brown sugar, flour, baking soda, salt, and rolled oats. Rub in the butter using your hands or a pastry blender to form a crumbly mixture. Press 2 cups of the mixture into the bottom of the prepared pan. Spread the jam to within 1/4 inch of the edge. Sprinkle the remaining crumb mixture over the top, and lightly press it into the jam.
3. Bake for 35 to 40 minutes in preheated oven, or until lightly browned. Allow to cool before cutting into bars.

Total: 45 mins

Servings: 4

Ingredients

- 4 teaspoons extra-virgin olive oil
- 1 large onion, chopped
- 1 medium fennel bulb, cored and chopped
- 5 cloves garlic, minced
- 1 teaspoon dried basil
- 1 (15 ounce) can cannellini or other white beans, rinsed
- 1 14-ounce can fire-roasted diced tomatoes
- 6 cups low-sodium vegetable broth
- ¾ cup quick-cooking barley
- 1 (5 ounce) package baby spinach (6 cups)
- ¼ cup grated Parmesan cheese
- ¼ teaspoon ground pepper

Directions

1. Heat oil in a Dutch oven over medium-high heat. Add onion, fennel, garlic, and basil; cook, stirring frequently, until tender and just beginning to brown, 6 to 8 minutes.
2. Mash 1/2 cup of the beans. Stir the mashed and whole beans, tomatoes, broth and barley into the pot. Bring to a boil over high heat. Reduce heat to medium and simmer, stirring occasionally, until the barley is tender, about 15 minutes. Stir in spinach and cook until wilted, about 1 minute. Remove from the heat and stir in cheese and pepper.

Prep: 30 mins

Cook: 35 mins

Additional: 25 mins

Total: 1 hr 30 mins

Servings: 12

Ingredients

CRUST:

- 1 cup gluten-free all-purpose flour
- ½ cup almond meal
- ½ teaspoon baking soda
- ¼ teaspoon salt
- 1 cup gluten-free rolled oats
- ½ cup packed light brown sugar
- ½ cup white sugar
- ½ cup unsalted butter, melted
- 2 teaspoons vanilla extract
- ¼ teaspoon almond extract (Optional)

APRICOT GINGER FILLING:

- ⅓ cup white sugar
- 1 tablespoon cornstarch
- 2 cups pitted and diced apricots
- 1 tablespoon diced fresh ginger

Directions

1. Preheat oven to 350 degrees F (175 degrees C). Grease an 8-inch baking dish and line with parchment paper; grease parchment paper.
2. Whisk flour, almond meal, baking soda, and salt together in a bowl. Add oats, brown sugar, and 1/2 cup white sugar; whisk to blend and break up clumps of brown sugar. Pour melted butter, vanilla extract, and almond extract over flour mixture; stir with a spatula until moistened.
3. Press 2/3 of the flour mixture into the bottom of the prepared baking dish to make the crust.
4. Whisk 1/3 cup white sugar and cornstarch together in a small bowl. Add apricots and ginger and toss to coat.
5. Spread apricot mixture over the crust. Sprinkle remaining 1/3 of the flour mixture on top.
6. Bake in the preheated oven until top is golden brown and crisp and filling is bubbling, 35 to 40 minutes. Cool completely before cutting into bars, about 25 minutes.

Prep: 15 mins

Cook: 30 mins

Total: 45 mins

Servings: 4

Ingredients

- 4 apples
- 1 cup rolled oats
- ¼ cup brown sugar
- 1 teaspoon ground cinnamon
- ¼ cup butter

Directions

1. Preheat oven to 350 degrees F (175 degrees C).
2. Core each apple making a large well in the center and arrange apples on a rimmed baking sheet.
3. Mix oats, brown sugar, and cinnamon together in a bowl; cut in butter until evenly combined. Spoon 1/4 of the oat mixture into each apple.
4. Bake in the preheated oven until apples are tender and filling is bubbling, about 30 minutes.

Total: 30 mins

Servings: 5

Ingredients

- 2 teaspoons plus 1 tablespoon extra-virgin olive oil, divided
- ½ cup carrot or diced red bell pepper
- 1 large boneless, skinless chicken breast (about 8 ounces), cut into quarters
- 1 large clove garlic, minced
- 5 cups reduced-sodium chicken broth
- 1 ½ teaspoons dried marjoram
- 6 ounces baby spinach, coarsely chopped
- 1 15-ounce can cannellini beans or great northern beans, rinsed
- ¼ cup grated Parmesan cheese
- ⅓ cup lightly packed fresh basil leaves
- Freshly ground pepper to taste
- ¾ cup plain or herbed multigrain croutons for garnish (optional)

Directions

1. Heat 2 teaspoons oil in a large saucepan or Dutch oven over medium-high heat. Add carrot (or bell pepper) and chicken; cook, turning the chicken and stirring frequently, until the chicken begins to brown, 3 to 4 minutes. Add garlic and cook, stirring, for 1 minute more. Stir in broth and marjoram; bring to a boil over high heat. Reduce the heat and simmer, stirring

occasionally, until the chicken is cooked through, about 5 minutes.

2. With a slotted spoon, transfer the chicken pieces to a clean cutting board to cool. Add spinach and beans to the pot and bring to a gentle boil. Cook for 5 minutes to blend the flavors.

3. Combine the remaining 1 tablespoon oil, Parmesan and basil in a food processor (a mini processor works well). Process until a coarse paste forms, adding a little water and scraping down the sides as necessary.

4. Cut the chicken into bite-size pieces. Stir the chicken and pesto into the pot. Season with pepper. Heat until hot. Garnish with croutons, if desired.

Total: 40 mins

Servings: 4

Ingredients

- 2 tablespoons extra-virgin olive oil
- 1 large onion, diced
- 1-3 teaspoons hot paprika, or to taste
- 2 14-ounce cans vegetable broth
- 4 medium plum tomatoes, diced
- 1 medium yellow summer squash, diced
- 2 cups diced cooked potatoes
- 1 ½ cups green beans, cut into 2-inch pieces
- 2 cups frozen spinach, (5 ounces)
- 2 tablespoons sherry vinegar, or red-wine vinegar
- 1/4 cup chopped fresh basil, or prepared pesto

Direction

1. Heat oil in a Dutch oven over medium heat. Add onion, cover and cook, stirring occasionally, until beginning to brown, about 6 minutes. Add paprika and cook, stirring, for 30 seconds. Add broth, tomatoes, squash, potatoes and beans; bring to a boil. Reduce heat to a simmer and cook, stirring occasionally, until the vegetables are just tender, about 12 minutes. Stir in spinach and vinegar; continue cooking until heated through, 2 to 4 minutes more. Ladle soup into bowls and top with fresh basil or a dollop of pesto.

Prep: 10 mins

Cook: 20 mins

Total: 30 mins

Servings: 6

Yield: 12 pancakes

Ingredients

- 1 ½ cups old-fashioned oatmeal
- 1 ½ cups whole wheat flour
- 2 teaspoons baking soda
- 1 teaspoon baking powder
- ½ teaspoon salt
- 1 ½ cups buttermilk
- 1 cup milk
- ¼ cup vegetable oil
- 1 egg
- ⅓ cup sugar
- 3 tablespoons chopped walnuts (Optional)

Directions

1. Grind the oats in a blender or food processor until fine. In a large bowl, combine ground oats, whole wheat flour, baking soda, baking powder, and salt.
2. In another bowl, combine buttermilk, milk, oil, egg, and sugar with an electric mixer until smooth. Mix wet ingredients into dry with a few swift strokes. Stir in nuts, if desired.

3. Lightly oil a skillet or griddle, and preheat it to medium heat. Ladle 1/3 cup of the batter onto the hot skillet; cook the pancakes for 2 to 4 minutes per side, or until brown.

Prep: 20 mins

Additional: 2 hrs

Total: 2 hrs 20 mins

Servings: 48

Ingredients

- 4 cups regular rolled oats
- 1 ¼ cups white sugar
- ½ cup unsweetened cocoa powder
- 1 cup butter or margarine, softened
- 2 tablespoons strong coffee
- 1 teaspoon vanilla extract
- 2 (1 ounce) squares unsweetened baking chocolate, melted
- ⅓ cup coconut flakes

Directions

1. Mix the oats, sugar, and cocoa together in a bowl. Add the butter, and use your hands to mix the ingredients together to make a thick dough. Mix in the coffee, vanilla, and chocolate until thoroughly blended.
2. Place the coconut flakes in a small bowl. Pinch off small amounts of dough and roll between your hands to make small balls, about 1-1/2 inches in diameter. Roll the balls in the coconut flakes. Balls are ready to eat, or may be refrigerated 2 hours to become firmer.

Prep: 20 mins

Additional: 30 mins

Total: 50 mins

Servings: 8

Ingredients

- ¼ cup lemon juice
- 1 teaspoon kosher salt
- 1 teaspoon seasoned salt
- ¼ teaspoon chili powder
- ½ cup olive oil
- 1 cup hot water
- ¾ cup bulgur
- 2 cups chopped fresh flat-leaf parsley
- 1 cup diced tomato
- ½ cup diced green bell pepper
- ½ cup peeled and diced cucumber
- 6 green onions, thinly sliced
- 1 tablespoon chopped fresh mint

Directions

1. Whisk lemon juice, kosher salt, seasoned salt, and chili powder together in a bowl. Slowly drizzle in olive oil while whisking rapidly until dressing is thick and creamy.
2. Pour hot water over bulgur in a bowl; let soak until water is absorbed and bulgur is soft, about 30 minutes.

3. Mix parsley, tomato, green bell pepper, cucumber, green onions, and mint together in a large bowl. Add bulgur; toss to combine.
4. Drizzle dressing over bulgur mixture; toss to coat.

Prep: 10 mins

Cook: 5 mins

Additional: 1 hr 40 mins

Total: 1 hr 55 mins

Servings: 8

Ingredients

- 1 cup chicken stock
- 1 cup bulgur wheat
- 1 (15.5 ounce) can black beans, rinsed and drained
- 1 (15.5 ounce) can whole kernel corn, drained
- 1 pint grape tomatoes, halved
- ¼ cup diced green bell pepper
- ¼ cup diced red onion
- 1 fresh red chile pepper

DRESSING:

- ⅓ cup lime juice
- ⅓ cup chopped fresh cilantro
- 1 tablespoon grated lime zest
- 2 tablespoons honey
- 1 tablespoon white wine vinegar
- ½ tablespoon minced garlic
- 1 teaspoon ground cumin
- 1 teaspoon salt
- ½ tablespoon extra-virgin olive oil
- 1 large avocado

Directions

1. Bring chicken stock to a boil in a medium saucepan over high heat. Remove from heat and pour in bulgur wheat. Stir to mix well, then cover and let sit for 30 minutes.
2. Meanwhile, combine black beans, corn, tomatoes, green pepper, and red onion in a medium salad bowl. Halve chile pepper and scrape out seeds; reserve for dressing. Dice chile and mix into the bowl.
3. Place chile seeds, lime juice, cilantro, lime zest, honey, vinegar, garlic, cumin, and salt in a bowl. Slowly pour in olive oil, whisking until dressing is combined.
4. Uncover bulgur and let cool, about 10 minutes. Add to the vegetable mixture and toss to combine. Pour in dressing and toss to coat. Cover salad and refrigerate for at least 1 hour.
5. Dice avocado and toss into the salad before serving.

Active: 30 mins

Total: 40 mins

Servings: 8

Ingredients

- 1 cup dried chickpeas
- 1 large clove garlic, chopped
- ¾ teaspoon salt, divided
- 2 cups whole-milk plain yogurt
- 2 tablespoons tahini
- 1 tablespoon extra-virgin olive oil plus 1/2 teaspoon, divided
- 3 tablespoons pine nuts
- 1 whole-wheat pita bread, split
- Chopped fresh parsley for garnish

Directions

1. Place chickpeas in a large bowl. Add enough cold water to cover by 3 inches and let soak for 8 to 24 hours. (Alternatively, place chickpeas in a large saucepan and cover with 3 inches cold water. Bring to a boil and cook for 2 minutes. Remove from the heat. Let stand for 1 hour.)
2. Drain the chickpeas, transfer to a large saucepan and add water to cover by 2 inches. Bring to a boil over high heat, reduce to a simmer and cook until very tender, about 30 minutes.
3. Meanwhile, preheat oven to 400 degrees F.

4. Using a fork, mash garlic with 1/4 teaspoon salt to make a paste. Combine in a medium bowl with yogurt, tahini, 1 tablespoon oil and 1/4 teaspoon salt. Set aside.
5. Heat the remaining 1/2 teaspoon oil and pine nuts in a small skillet over medium heat. Cook, stirring frequently, until lightly browned, 2 to 3 minutes. Transfer to a small bowl.
6. Place pita halves on the oven rack and bake until crisp and golden, turning once, 6 to 8 minutes total. Let cool slightly then break into pieces.
7. Drain the chickpeas, reserving 1/4 cup cooking water. Return the chickpeas and the 1/4 cup water to the pot; stir in the remaining 1/4 teaspoon salt. Transfer the chickpeas to a shallow serving dish. Top with the reserved yogurt sauce, pita pieces and pine nuts. Garnish with parsley, if desired. Serve immediately.

Active: 25 mins

Total: 25 mins

Servings: 4

Ingredients

- 4 (5 ounce) salmon fillets (fresh or frozen, thawed), skin and pin bones removed
- ¼ cup nonfat plain Greek yogurt
- 1 small shallot, finely chopped
- 2 tablespoons finely chopped fresh Italian parsley
- 2 teaspoons cider vinegar
- 1 teaspoon prepared horseradish
- 1 teaspoon Dijon mustard
- ¼ teaspoon sweet paprika plus 1/8 teaspoon, divided
- ⅛ teaspoon garlic powder plus 1/4 teaspoon, divided
- Pinch of salt plus 1/4 teaspoon, divided
- Pinch of ground pepper plus 1/8 teaspoon, divided
- 3 teaspoons olive oil, divided

Directions

1. Bring fish to room temperature by letting it stand on the counter for 15 minutes.
2. Meanwhile, whisk together yogurt, shallot, parsley, vinegar, horseradish, mustard, 1/4 tsp. paprika, 1/8 tsp. garlic powder, and a pinch each of salt and pepper in a small bowl. Cover and refrigerate until ready to use.
3. Pat both sides of the fish dry with a paper towel. Brush both sides with 2 tsp. oil. Season both sides evenly with

the remaining 1/4 tsp. each salt and garlic powder, and 1/8 tsp. each paprika and pepper.

4. Heat the remaining 1 tsp. oil in a large nonstick skillet over medium-high heat. When hot, add the fish, skinned-side up. Cook, pressing down on the fish with a spatula, but otherwise not moving the fillets, until the undersides are golden brown, about 5 minutes.

5. Using the spatula, very carefully flip the fillets. Continue cooking, without moving, until the undersides are golden brown and the fish is opaque and just beginning to flake, another 2 to 3 minutes. Serve immediately, with the remoulade.

Active: 20 mins

Total: 25 mins

Servings: 4

Ingredients

- 2 tablespoons extra-virgin olive oil
- 4 cups baby spinach, chopped (about 5 ounces)
- 4 cloves garlic, sliced
- 2 cups canned crushed tomatoes
- 1 (15 ounce) can no-salt-added chickpeas, rinsed
- ¼ cup heavy cream
- ½ teaspoon salt
- 4 large eggs
- 1 tablespoon chopped fresh thyme
- ½ teaspoon ground pepper

Directions

1. Heat oil in large skillet over medium heat. Add spinach and garlic. Cook, stirring, until the spinach has wilted and the garlic is beginning to brown, about 2 minutes.
2. Reduce heat to medium-low. Add tomatoes, chickpeas, cream and salt. Adjust heat to maintain a simmer. Crack an egg into a small bowl, taking care not to break the yolk. Make a well in the sauce roughly large enough to hold the egg and slip it in so that the yolk and most of the white is contained (some white may spread out). Repeat with the remaining eggs, evenly spacing them around the pan. Sprinkle the sauce with thyme; cover and cook until the eggs reach desired doneness, 6 to 8

minutes for medium-set. Remove from the heat and sprinkle with pepper.

Active: 45 mins

Total: 45 mins

Servings: 12

Ingredients

PEA PUREE

- 2 cups fresh shelled English peas (from about 2 pounds unshelled) or frozen
- 1 cup fennel fronds
- ½ cup extra-virgin olive oil
- ½ cup packed fresh mint
- 1 stalk green garlic, chopped
- 2 tablespoons lemon juice
- ½ teaspoon kosher salt
- ¼ teaspoon ground pepper

TOASTS

- 6 1/2-inch-thick slices pain au levain or whole-wheat country bread, cut in half
- 1 tablespoon extra-virgin olive oil plus 2 teaspoons, divided
- 2 lemons
- 1 small fennel bulb, halved, cored and thinly sliced
- Pinch each of kosher salt & pepper
- 12 sardines and/or anchovies
- ¼ cup fresh mint, cut into pieces or torn

Directions

1. To prepare puree: Bring a large saucepan of water to a boil. Set a bowl of ice water near the stove. Cook peas in the boiling water until tender, 2 to 4 minutes. Transfer to the ice bath until cold, 1 to 2 minutes. Remove the ice, then drain the peas in a colander. Let them stand until well drained, shaking the colander a few times, about 2 minutes.

2. Transfer the peas to a food processor and add fennel fronds, 1/2 cup each oil and mint, green garlic, lemon juice, 1/2 teaspoon salt and 1/4 teaspoon pepper. Puree until slightly chunky, scraping down the sides once or twice.

3. To prepare toasts: Position a rack in top third of oven; preheat broiler to high.

4. Place bread on a baking sheet and brush both sides with 1 tablespoon oil. Broil until browned and crisp, about 2 minutes per side. Let cool for 5 minutes.

5. Juice 1 lemon. Toss fennel with the juice, the remaining 2 teaspoons oil and salt and pepper. Spread 2 tablespoons of the pea puree on each toast. Divide the fennel among the toasts, lightly pressing it into the puree. Top each with a sardine (or anchovy). Top with mint. Cut the remaining lemon into wedges and serve with the toasts.

25. No-Bake Berry Cheesecake Bars

Active: 20 mins

Total: 2 hrs 20 mins

Servings: 16

Ingredients

- 7 ounces graham crackers, broken into large pieces
- ½ cup toasted pecans
- ¼ teaspoon salt
- ⅓ cup canola oil
- 2 (8 ounce) packages reduced-fat cream cheese, softened
- 2 cups nonfat plain Greek yogurt
- ⅔ cup confectioners' sugar
- 1 teaspoon lemon zest
- 1 tablespoon lemon juice
- 5 cups fresh berries

Directions

1. Pulse graham crackers, pecans and salt in a food processor until finely ground. With the motor running, drizzle in oil, then pulse to combine. Press into a 9-by-13-inch baking dish.
2. Add cream cheese, yogurt, confectioners' sugar, lemon zest and lemon juice to the food processor. Puree until smooth, about 1 minute. Dollop the mixture over the crust, then gently spread into an even layer. Cover and refrigerate until cold, at least 2 hours and up to 1 day.
3. To serve, top with berries and cut into 16 squares.

Prep: 15 mins

Cook: 42 mins

Total: 57 mins

Servings: 4

Ingredients

- 4 red bell peppers, halved lengthwise and seeded
- 1 cup water
- ½ cup bulgur
- 1 (24 ounce) jar tomato sauce, or more to taste
- 2 cups arugula
- 1 cup corn kernels
- ½ cup garbanzo beans, drained
- ½ cup lima beans, drained
- ½ cup black beans, rinsed and drained
- ½ cup kidney beans, rinsed and drained
- 1 teaspoon salt
- ½ teaspoon paprika
- ½ teaspoon dried basil
- ½ teaspoon dried oregano

Directions

1. Preheat oven to 350 degrees F (175 degrees C). Line a 9x11-inch baking pan with aluminum foil. Arrange bell pepper halves in the baking pan.
2. Bring water and bulgur to a boil in a small saucepan. Cover and simmer until bulgur is tender, 12 to 15 minutes. Drain excess water.

3. Combine bulgur, tomato sauce, arugula, corn kernels, garbanzo beans, lima beans, black beans, kidney beans, salt, paprika, basil, and oregano in a large bowl. Fill each bell pepper half generously with bulgur mixture.
4. Bake in the preheated oven until bubbly and hot, 25 to 30 minutes.

Prep: 25 mins

Cook: 15 mins

Additional: 5 mins

Total: 45 mins

Servings: 7

Ingredients

- 1 ¾ cups water
- 1 cup red lentils
- ¾ cup fine bulgur (cracked wheat)
- 3 tablespoons olive oil
- 7 spring onions, finely chopped, or more to taste
- 1 ½ tablespoons tomato paste
- ½ bunch parsley, minced
- ½ lemon, juiced
- 1 ½ teaspoons red pepper flakes
- 1 teaspoon ground cumin
- 1 teaspoon salt

Directions

1. Combine water and red lentils in a saucepan; bring to a boil. Reduce heat and simmer until water is absorbed, about 10 minutes. Stir in bulgur and remove saucepan from heat. Cover and let stand until bulgur absorbs the residual moisture, about 5 minutes.
2. Heat olive oil in a skillet over medium heat. Cook and stir spring onions until softened, 3 to 5 minutes. Stir in tomato paste; cook for 2 to 3 minutes.

3. Combine red lentil mixture and onion mixture in a large bowl. Add parsley, lemon juice, red pepper flakes, cumin, and salt; knead by hand until evenly distributed.
4. Shape mixture into small logs or round balls and arrange on a plate. Cover with plastic wrap to prevent the tops from drying out before serving.

Prep: 30 mins

Cook: 48 mins

Total: 1 hr 18 mins

Servings: 10

Ingredients

- 2 cups water
- 1 cup bulgur
- 1 tablespoon olive oil
- 2 cups shredded carrots
- 1 large onion, chopped
- 1 green bell pepper, chopped
- 1 red bell pepper, chopped
- ½ jalapeno pepper, seeded and minced
- 2 cloves garlic, minced, or more to taste
- 5 cups reduced-sodium tomato juice
- 2 (16 ounce) cans kidney beans
- 2 (16 ounce) cans black beans
- 1 (28 ounce) can petite diced tomatoes, undrained
- 1 (8 ounce) can low-sodium tomato sauce
- 2 tablespoons chili powder
- 2 tablespoons taco seasoning
- 1 ½ teaspoons ground cumin
- ¼ teaspoon cayenne pepper
- ¼ teaspoon ground black pepper

Directions

1. Pour water and bulgur into a saucepan. Bring to a boil; cover and simmer until tender, 12 to 15 minutes. Drain off excess water.
2. Heat olive oil in a large pot over medium heat. Add carrots, onions, green bell pepper, red bell pepper, and jalapeno pepper; cook and stir until softened and starting to brown, 5 to 10 minutes. Stir in garlic; cook and stir until fragrant, 1 to 2 minutes.
3. Stir cooked bulgur, tomato juice, kidney beans, black beans, diced tomatoes, tomato sauce, chili powder, taco seasoning, cumin, cayenne, and pepper into the pot. Bring to a boil; reduce heat and simmer until flavors combine, 20 to 30 minutes.

Prep: 20 mins

Cook: 30 mins

Additional: 20 mins

Total: 1 hr 10 mins

Servings: 6

Ingredients

SALAD:

- 4 cups boiling water
- 1 cube vegetable bouillon
- 1 cup dry lentils
- 1 cup bulgur
- 2 cups boiling water
- 1 cup minced fresh parsley
- ½ cup minced sweet onion

DRESSING:

- ¼ cup chicken broth
- 2 tablespoons red wine vinegar
- 1 tablespoon cider vinegar
- 1 tablespoon Dijon mustard
- 1 tablespoon olive oil
- 2 cloves garlic, minced
- 1 teaspoon dried oregano
- ½ teaspoon Worcestershire sauce
- ½ teaspoon dried basil
- ¼ teaspoon ground cumin
- ¼ teaspoon salt, or to taste

- ⅛ teaspoon hot pepper sauce
- freshly ground black pepper to taste
- ½ cup thinly sliced scallions

Directions

1. Combine 4 cups boiling water and bouillon cube in a saucepan until dissolved; add lentils and cook over medium heat until lentils are tender, about 30 minutes. Remove saucepan from heat and let stand for 10 minutes. Drain excess water.
2. Put bulgur in a heat-proof bowl; pour in 2 cups boiling water. Let mixture stand until bulgur has absorbed most of the water and is tender, about 10 minutes. Drain excess water.
3. Combine lentils, bulgur, onion, and parsley in a large bowl.
4. Mix chicken broth, red wine vinegar, cider vinegar, mustard, olive oil, garlic, oregano, Worcestershire sauce, basil, cumin, salt, hot sauce, and black pepper in a jar. Cover jar with tight-fitting lid and shake until dressing is well-mixed. Pour dressing over lentil mixture and mix well; top with scallions.

Prep: 30 mins

Cook: 55 mins

Total: 1 hr 25 mins

Servings: 8

Ingredients

- ¾ cup bulgur
- ¾ cup boiling water
- 2 ½ tablespoons vegetable oil
- 2 cups sliced onions
- 4 cloves garlic, minced
- 6 cups thickly sliced zucchini
- ½ teaspoon dried oregano
- ½ teaspoon dried basil
- ½ teaspoon dried marjoram
- ⅛ teaspoon ground black pepper
- 2 eggs
- 1 cup grated feta cheese
- 1 cup cottage cheese
- ½ cup chopped fresh parsley
- 2 tablespoons tomato paste
- 1 tablespoon tamari
- 1 cup grated Cheddar cheese
- 2 medium tomatoes, thinly sliced
- 1 ½ tablespoons sesame seeds (Optional)

Directions

1. Place bulgur in a bowl and cover with boiling water. Cover and set aside until water is absorbed.
2. Preheat the oven to 350 degrees F (175 degrees C). Grease a 9-inch square casserole dish.
3. Meanwhile, heat oil in a large skillet over medium heat. Add onions and garlic and cook until just translucent, 3 to 5 minutes. Add zucchini, oregano, basil, marjoram, and black pepper. Cook until zucchini is tender but not falling apart, about 5 minutes more.
4. Beat eggs lightly in a bowl. Add feta cheese and cottage cheese.
5. Add parsley, tomato paste, and tamari to the bowl with the bulgur and mix well.
6. Layer bulgur mixture, zucchini mixture, cheese mixture, Cheddar cheese, and tomato into the prepared casserole dish. Sprinkle sesame seeds on top. Cover with aluminum foil.
7. Bake in the preheated oven until bubbly, about 45 minutes.